# KetoCook: Ketogenic Diet for Weight Loss

## The Definitive Beginner's Guide to Weight Loss with the Ketogenic Diet

*Ben Plus Publishing*

# Table of Contents

# Introduction

**Ketogenic diets** have been proven to be therapeutic. In fact, it is recommended as one of the possible treatments for epilepsy. But what is a ketogenic diet?

Nowadays, when you read or hear about **ketogenic diets**, it is usually related to or used for weight loss. However, it's really an old practice that's been around for hundreds of years. This diet is in fact not a product of modern discovery.

## What Is a Ketogenic Diet?

This diet is both a dietary medical therapy as well as a lifestyle choice with the aim of burning the excess fat from off the body. A ketogenic diet is actually a type of low carbohydrate diet. It was originally intended in modern times as a treatment for refractory epilepsy among children.

The main idea behind this dietary therapy is to make the body make metabolic adjustments. The diet makes the body perform changes in its processes insomuch that it will make use of fats as the main source of fuel or source of energy rather than carbohydrates. In today's diet, the body processes carbohydrates in food to make glucose (a type of simple sugar).

Glucose is then transported to the entire body, especially where it is needed. It acts like fuel that the body burns in order to get energy. Glucose is actually an important nutrient for a lot of functions in the brain.

Doing that is like starving the brain of its primary energy source; but isn't that dangerous? The answer is that it isn't really detrimental to the health of the patient. Take note that glucose from carbs is not the only energy source or fuel that the brain can use.

The body, especially the brain, only uses glucose simply because there is plenty of supply. That is basically due to the fact that our diets today is heavy in carbohydrates (a lot of it are actually processed carbs). Unfortunately, today's diet actually supplies the body with too much glucose.

When there is too much glucose, the body doesn't make use of it all. Of course, the human metabolism is well-designed and it's actually really smart. Since there is an excess of carbs/glucose then the body stores it in the form of body fat.

What a low carb ketogenic diet does is to force the body to reverse the process. It's obvious that many of the dieters today have an excess of body fat. There's really no point in taking in more carbs since it only produces more added weight and body fat.

The secret behind this kind of low carb diet is found in the way the liver operates. Ketogenic diets lower the carb intake of the individual. This condition will then signal to the body that carbs or glucose is now in short supply.

The way the human metabolism is designed, it will make a switch in the primary fuel or energy source. Since the former primary fuel source is now scarce, it will turn to fats as the main energy source of the body. That is why the fat was stored in the first place (they act as some sort of energy reserve). In the case of an obese dieter undergoing a **ketogenic diet**, there is a huge supply of body fat that the entire body can use.

The liver will start to make use of the stored body fat and turn it into fatty acids. During this process, ketone bodies are also produced. This byproduct is the reason behind the name of the diet. You can live on a really low carb diet if your body is in ketosis; your liver will start to produce those ketone bodies that will be used by the brain.

The ketone bodies that were produced from converting body fat are passed into the brain through the blood stream. The brain then uses them as its energy source in order to perform its functions. Medical experts have observed that as the level of ketone bodies flowing in the blood rises, the number of epileptic seizures tends to decrease.

Given the effects of this diet, it is easy to see the two main benefits that can be garnered from it. The first one is that more body fat is metabolized naturally. The second one is that it helps to prevent seizures in epilepsy patients. It is both a weight loss technique and a natural epilepsy treatment.

Since the main thrust of this work is not about using ketosis to treat epilepsy, the content you will find later on mainly focuses on its use as a weight loss tool. Remember that this diet is not only a therapy for epilepsy patients. In fact it can also be used as a medical treatment for obesity.

# The History of Low Calorie and Ketogenic Diets

History points to the fact that the diet of human beings didn't always contain a lot of carbohydrates. In fact, human beings only increased their carb intake after man learned general agriculture thus understanding how to cultivate plants and grain for food. Human beings are genetically attuned to low carbohydrate diets.

This means that the human body is naturally adapted to a diet that doesn't necessarily have a lot of carbs. After man learned agriculture, human beings began to adapt to a carb rich diet. And since human beings can adapt easily to survive, man has learned to thrive on such high carb diets with other nutrients and food sources taking a back seat.

There is fossil evidence dating back to the Paleolithic era that shows that human beings have subsisted on low carb diets for a time. It should be remembered that during this era, human beings hunted for food. The habit of gathering fruits and other plant based food cannot sustain a high carb diet. There is also evidence that other early human species (such as Neanderthals) are primarily carnivorous and not herbivorous or omnivorous.

Of course, there are opposing views to what the archaeological evidence actually means. People interpret evidence in a variety of ways. But it cannot be denied that man only mass produced grains and other carbohydrate sources later in history.

In the 19th century, doctors used ketogenic diets and low carbohydrate diets as the main treatment for patients with diabetes. An example of which is Dr. John Rollo's treatment of two diabetes mellitus cases using a low carb diet. Of course, other similar diets and recipes came about following the same vein such as James Salisbury's Salisbury Steak introduced in 1888.

Other modern low carb and ketogenic diets include Richard Mackarness' diet (1958), Stillman Diet (1967), Air Force Diet (1960), and the popular Atkins Diet. A second and modified version of the Atkins Diet was introduced in the 1990s. The Zone Diet and other low carb diets were also introduced during the past couple of decades but these diets never escaped controversy and criticism in spite of their popularity at the time.

# Why are Ketogenic Diets and Low Carb Diets Better than Low Fat Diets?

A meta-analysis conducted by the British Journal of Nutrition in 2013 reports that low carbohydrate diets and ketogenic diets can help people achieve greater weight loss in the long term. Furthermore, the Journal of the International Society of Sports Nutrition released a paper that stressed two important points, mainly the following:

(1) Diets that have a high fat content are the not the main cause of obesity. This means that even if you reduce the amount of fat you eat each day this will have very little effect on your weight loss efforts.

(2) Low fat diets that are marketed nowadays cannot demonstrate that they are any better than control diets. This means they barely provide any weight loss results even if you strictly follow diets that restrict the amount of fat you consume. Many people frown at restrictive diets nowadays

The usual formula for weight loss is that the calories that a person uses or spends should be greater than the calories that he takes in. If both are equal then, theoretically, there should be no change in the body composition of the subject. However, in today's modern western diets (and this phenomenon is also showing up in other parts of the world as well), most people take in more calories than they are using.

Where do you think does most of the caloric load come from? They don't come from fat but they are actually from carbohydrates (both liquid carbs and solid carbs). A lot of energy (in the form of calories) is ingested by people nowadays given their diets but very little is spent in the form of physical effort; a byproduct of the lifestyle of many today.

This is one of the reasons why low carb diets and ketogenic diets are more effective in the long run. But that is not the only advantage that these diets provide where weight loss is concerned. Another trump card that these diets have in store is their effect on a person's metabolism including the hormonal changes associated with it.

You may think that the trick of switching from using carbs to fat as the primary energy source of the body is a short lived feat; then you better think again. Studies show that low carb diets can reduce the level of insulin in the blood and thereby increasing the level of glucagons. When that happens gluconeogenesis occurs instead of glycolysis.

Take note that gluconeogenesis is a body process that promotes the natural consumption or use of energy. In this process gluconeogenic amino acids (coming from fat) is processed and transformed by the body into glucose. This process requires the body to dispose of the nitrogen content in the form of urea. Doing that will require more energy, this means that the body's metabolic processes are already working for you to burn off energy. That's like your body doing a workout on its own spending calories without making you go to the gym or do any exercises.

Now, the natural energy consuming metabolic processes do not end there. There are other processes in the conversion of fat into usable bodily energy that will eventually require the metabolism to do the workout for you. Another example of that is found in the body's turnover of protein.

Take note that most low carb diets as well as ketogenic diets prescribe the intake of more healthy fat and protein sources as energy replacements. The way the body transforms or makes use of proteins as an energy source also contributes to the natural calorie expenditure. In this way your metabolism is working for you to attain weight loss.

This bodily phenomenon was confirmed on February of 2002 by a study published in the Journal of the American College of Nutrition. This piece of research shows that postprandial thermogenesis can increase to as much as 100 percent on a high protein low fat diet. The results were compared to the effects of a high carbohydrate and low fat diet. Note that the test subjects of the said study were all healthy.

One final way in which a ketogenic diet or a low carb diet can work for you to lose weight is in its ability to increase the level of free fatty acids. If the level of free fatty acids increases in the body, it produces two effects: (1) uncoupling protein transcription and (2) peroxisomal beta oxidation. Uncoupling proteins result in the body's generation of heat. On the other hand, the beta oxidation process of fatty acids doesn't have a mechanism for energy conservation thus more energy is consumed and more heat is produced. The bottom line here is that more energy is spent and this leads to what experts call a metabolic inefficiency.

# Looking Beyond the Weight Loss Curtain

Losing weight per se is good but that is not the main thrust of any weight loss program. The big question in any diet or weight loss regimen is what components of weight loss are being dealt with. A person's weight is composed of many different things. You have to consider muscle mass as well as the amount of fat lost.

If one is gaining weight but is actually increasing muscle mass then that is not really an unhealthy weight gain. In fact, all things considered, when you increase muscle mass in any weight control routine, that is a good result. Your muscles actually contribute in long term calorie burn.

In the case of ketogenic diets, in order for you to really figure out if you are actually losing weight in a healthy way is when the amount of body fat is being reduced. Related to this was a study that was published way back in 1965 by Benoit and associates.

Their study observed the effects of a highly ketogenic diet (one that provided test subjects with only 1,000 kilo calories or about ten grams of carbohydrates per day). The test subjects only consumed that amount of carbohydrates for 10 straight days. Test subjects were seven males.

It was observed in that study that all seven test subjects experienced a weight loss of 600 grams per day. That translates to a six kilogram weight loss during the duration of the entire experiment. But the weight loss alone wasn't the only dramatic thing that was discovered.

It was also discovered that 97% of the weight that the test subjects lost was basically fat and not some other body component. That alone is a truly remarkable result. Such results cannot be achieved by undergoing low fat diets.

There are of course more recent studies that have tried to verify the results of that experiment. One example of which was conducted by MJ Sharman,

DM Love, and JS Volek in 2002. The study was also published in Nutrition and Metabolism (London) November 8, 2004 edition page 13. Their results pretty much resemble those achieved by Benoit in 1965.

Experts have concluded that weight loss using ketogenic diets are expected to be rapid. They also observed further that the process is also consistent, which means that the rate in which the weight is lost is pretty much even if measured on a regular or daily basis. The same experts agree that it is definitely an effective tool to lose weight.

The next question however is if this weight loss regimen is healthy. Losing 6 or more kilograms in a week is rather dramatic. Some may think that it may be detrimental to a person's health. The same experts who observed their test subjects report that the lost weight comes almost exclusively from fat stores in the body. They conclude that it is definitely a healthy weight loss.

But before you jump on a ketogenic diet, you should note that switching to one is not easy. Along with the positive successful reports come many test subjects who failed to comply with the requirements of such a diet.

It's effective but it is really hard to live up to it. It's not as easy as you may think it is. Another thing that should also be noted is the fact that many of the test subjects were healthy. Dieters who have other medical conditions like diabetes should first consult with their doctors if a **ketogenic diet** will be feasible for them. If it isn't then perhaps other low carb diets that aren't as taxing can be used as an alternative (i.e. not all low carb diets are ketogenic).

# Beginners' Ketogenic Diet Recipes

# Breakfast Ideas

# Lox and Avocado Crêpes

Prep Time: 10 minutes

Dehydrating Time: 7 - 10 hours

Servings: 2

## INGREDIENTS

4 - 6 oz smoked salmon

1 ripe avocado

1/2 lemon

1 sprig fresh dill

1 teaspoon sesame seeds (black or white)

*Crêpes*

1 young coconut (plus coconut water)

1/3 cup raw sunflower seeds

1/2 cup flax seeds

1/2 white ground pepper (or 1/4 teaspoon ground black pepper)

1/2 teaspoon Celtic sea salt

Water

## INSTRUCTIONS

1.  For *Crêpes*, add flax to food processor or high-speed blender. Process until finely ground, up to 5 minutes. Add sunflower seeds and process until finely ground, about 1 minute.

2. Remove flesh and water from young coconut. Add to processor with salt and pepper. Process until smooth batter forms, about 1 - 2 minutes. Add enough water to reach desired consistency.

3. Place parchment paper or dehydrator sheets on dehydrator trays.

4. Spread batter on prepared sheets. Place trays in dehydrator and set to 115 degrees F for 6 - 8 hours.

5. Remove trays from dehydrator. Remove *Crêpes* from parchment or dehydrator liners, flip, and place directly on dehydrator tray. Place trays back in dehydrator and continue dehydrating 1 - 2 hours, until surface is dry but *Crêpe* is still pliable.

6. Remove from dehydrator and cut into desired shape and size. Set aside.

7. Finely chop fresh dill. Cut avocado in half and remove pit. Slice flesh in peel.

8. Lay *Crêpes* flat and top with line of smoked salmon down center. Scoop portion of sliced avocado over smoked salmon. Sprinkle on chopped dill. Roll up *Crêpes* and transfer to serving dish.

9. Top *Crêpes* with squeeze of lemon juice and sprinkle on sesame seeds. Serve immediately.

# Turkey Jerky Bacon

Prep Time: 10 minutes*

Dehydrating Time: 4 - 8 hours

Servings: 4

INGREDIENTS

4 oz organic turkey (dark meat)

2 tablespoons coconut aminos (or liquid aminos)

2 tablespoons tamari (or liquid aminos or coconut aminos)

1 tablespoon lemon juice (or raw apple cider vinegar)

1 tablespoons Celtic sea salt

1/2 teaspoon garlic powder

1/2 teaspoon onion powder

1/2 teaspoon smoked paprika

Pinch cayenne pepper

INSTRUCTIONS

1. Prepare two sheet parchment. Lay one on cutting board.
2. Cut turkey into 1/4 inch strips and lay in single layer on parchment. Pound with tenderizing side of kitchen mallet. Cover turkey with second parchment sheet, then pound with flat side of tenderizing mallet to 1/8 inch thickness.
3. *Place turkey strips in medium mixing bowl or shallow dish. Add coconut aminos, tamari, lemon juice, salt and spices. Mix well to coat. Cover and place in refrigerator for 8 hours, or overnight.

4. Remove turkey from refrigerator and lay in single layer on dehydrator trays. Place trays in dehydrator and set to 120 degrees F for 4 - 8 hours.

5. After 4 hours dehydrating time, remove trays from dehydrator and test turkey by bending. If it cracks, remove and serve immediately. Or store in airtight container.

6. If still flexible, place back in dehydrator and continue dehydrating up to 4 hours, or until desired texture is achieved.

# Stone-wrought Coop

Prep time: 5 minutes

Cook time: 3-6 minutes

INGREDIENTS

2 cage-free eggs

1 small onion

1 clove garlic

½ red bell pepper

1 tbsp extra virgin olive oil

¼ tsp smoked paprika

¼ tsp ground black pepper

INSTRUCTIONS

1. Finely chop onion, garlic and red bell pepper.
2. Pour extra virgin olive oil into a pan over medium heat.
3. Crack eggs and pour into a small bowl. Combine with onion, garlic and red bell pepper and whisk until mixed together.
4. Pour contents of bowl into pan and add smoked paprika and ground black pepper. Scramble until desired doneness. Serve.

# Ancient Egg Muffins

Prep time: 5 minutes

Cook time: 15-20 minutes

## INGREDIENTS

1 tbsp olive oil

1 tbsp coconut oil

6 cage-free eggs

1 onion

½ yellow bell pepper

½ red bell pepper

¼ tsp ground black pepper

¼ tsp Celtic sea salt

## INSTRUCTIONS

1. Preheat oven to 350. Whisk all 6 eggs in a bowl. Chop the onion and bell pepper into small pieces.
2. In a pan, combine olive oil with onion over medium-high heat for 2 minutes. Add peppers and cook another 2 minutes.
3. Remove onion/peppers from heat and let cool a few minutes. Combine them with the eggs. Add the Celtic sea salt and ground black pepper and mix.
4. Coat a muffin pan with the coconut oil. Fill each muffin cup with the egg/pepper/onion mix. Do not fill a muffin cup more than ¾ full.

5. Place the pan in the oven and bake 10-15 minutes, removing the pan from the oven when the tops of the muffins get fluffy and golden brown.

6. Remove the muffins from the pan and serve.

# Sizzled Chicken Wraps

Prep time: 5 minutes

Cook time: 3 minutes

INGREDIENTS

4 slices of chicken deli meat

1 tbsp olive oil

1 small onion

1 red bell pepper

1 avocado

¼ tsp garlic powder

INSTRUCTIONS

1. Remove the nut from the avocado and mash it into a paste. Chop the pepper and onion into small pieces.
2. Combine the garlic powder, pepper and onion in the bowl with the avocado and mix well.
3. Add the olive oil in a pan over low heat and heat the chicken mildly, turning frequently, for 3 minutes.
4. Remove the chicken from heat and place ¼ of the avocado/pepper/onion mixture onto each piece.
5. Wrap the chicken up into tubes and serve.

# Green Monster Kale and Poached Eggs

Prep time: 10 minutes

Cook time: 12 minutes

## INGREDIENTS

1 handful kale

2 cage-free eggs

1 small onion

1 clove garlic

1 tbsp extra virgin olive oil

¼ tsp ground black pepper

1 tsp low-sodium horseradish (optional)

## INSTRUCTIONS

1. Chop the onion and mince the garlic. De-stem and wash the kale. Leaving a bit of water on the kale is ideal.

2. In a saucepan, add 1 tbsp extra virgin olive oil over medium heat. Add onion and cook until it begins to lose its opaqueness, about 5 minutes.

3. Add kale to saucepan and cover until kale is soft and green, about 5 minutes. Add garlic and stir, then cook another 2 minutes and remove from heat.

4. Fill a saucepan half full of water. Bring the water to a boil, then reduce heat below a boil and hold it there.

5. One by one, crack the eggs into a small cup or bowl and, with the lip of the cup or bowl close to the water's surface, dump the egg

into the water. If necessary, nudge the eggwhites closer to the yolks to keep them together.

6. Once all the eggs are in the water, remove the pan from heat and cover it. Let sit for 4 minutes until all eggs are cooked, then remove eggs from pan.

7. Place the greens on a plate and the two eggs on top of the greens. Top with horseradish if desired. Serve.

# Lunch Ideas

## Mexican Tomato Soup

Prep Time: 35 minutes

Servings: 2

INGREDIENTS

*Shrimp*

10 - 12 large shrimp

1 - 1 1/2 cups lemon juice (about 8 lemons)

1/2 jalapeño pepper

*Gazpacho*

2 cups tomato juice (about 4 large tomatoes)

2 plum tomatoes

1/2 red bell pepper

1/2 red onion

1/2 cucumber

Small bunch fresh cilantro

2 garlic cloves

2 tablespoons raw apple cider vinegar(optional)

2 tablespoons raw oil (coconut, walnut, almond, sesame, etc.) (optional)

1 teaspoon ground black pepper

1 teaspoon Celtic sea salt

INSTRUCTIONS

1. For *Shrimp*, Peel, devein and remove tails from shrimp. Mince jalapeño and juice lemons. Add to small bowl and mix. Shrimp should be completely covered in lemon juice. Place in refrigerator for 30 minutes, or until shrimp are opaque.

2. For Gazpacho, juice large tomatoes in juicer. Or add to food processor or high-speed blender and process, then strain into medium mixing bowl.

3. Peel cucumber and seed. Seed plum tomatoes. Seed, stem and vein bell peppers. Peel onion and garlic. Dice veggies and onion, and mince garlic. Add to tomato juice.

4. Add salt, pepper, vinegar and oil (optional). Mix well, then place in refrigerator.

5. Chop cilantro and set aside.

6. Remove shrimp from refrigerator and drain lemon juice and jalapeños. Rinse if desired.

7. Mix shrimp into tomato mixture. Pour into serving bowls and top with chopped cilantro. Serve chilled.

# Texas Chili

Prep Time: 10 minutes*

Servings: 2

INGREDIENTS

5 - 6 plum tomatoes

1/2 teaspoon dried cumin

1/4 teaspoon chili powder

1/4 teaspoon onion powder

1/4 teaspoon garlic powder

1 teaspoon fresh oregano leaves  (or 1/4 teaspoon dried oregano)

1/2 teaspoon ground black pepper

1/4 teaspoon cayenne pepper or red pepper flakes (optional)

1  teaspoon Celtic sea salt

1 teaspoon chia seed (or flax seed)

1/2 cup raw cashews

Water

INSTRUCTIONS

1.  *Soak raw cashews in enough water to cover overnight in refrigerator. Drain and rinse. Set aside.

2.  Grind chia or flax in food processor or  high-speed blender. Set aside.

3.  Juice tomatoes. Or add to food processor or high-speed blender and process. Add enough water to reach desired consistency, if necessary. Then strain.

4. Add tomato juice, ground chia or flax, 1/2 of soaked cashews, salt, pepper and spices to blender. Process until smooth, about 1 - 2 minutes.
5. Stir in remaining soaked cashews.
6. Pour into serving bowls and serve immediately.

# Creamy "Cheese" and Broccoli Soup

Prep Time: 10 minutes*

Servings: 2

## INGREDIENTS

1 1/2 - 2 cups broccoli florets

1 red bell pepper

1 garlic clove

1/4 cup raw oil (coconut, walnut, almond, sesame, etc.)

1 cup nutritional yeast

1 tablespoon coconut aminos (or tamari)

1 tablespoon onion powder

1/2 teaspoon Celtic sea salt

1/4 teaspoon ground white pepper (or ground black pepper)

2 cups raw cashews

Water

## INSTRUCTIONS

1. * Soak raw cashews in enough water to cover at least 2 hours, or overnight in refrigerator. Drain and rinse. Set aside.
2. Chop broccoli florets into pieces and set aside.
3. Seed and vein bell pepper. Peel garlic. Add to food processor or high-speed blender with soaked cashews, nutritional yeast, coconut aminos, salt, pepper and enough water to process until smooth, about 2 - 3 minutes.
4. Pour into serving bowl and top with broccoli. Serve immediately.

# Caesar Salad

Prep Time: 10 minutes

Servings: 1

INGREDIENTS

2 cups chopped romaine lettuce

*Almond Parmesan*

1/4 cup raw almonds

1 teaspoon raw apple cider vinegar

1 teaspoon nutritional yeast (optional)

1/4 teaspoon garlic powder

1/4 teaspoon onion powder

1/4 teaspoon dried oregano

1/4 teaspoon Celtic sea salt

*Raw Caesar Dressing*

2 tablespoons raw cashews (or raw sunflower seeds)

2 tablespoons raw sunflower seeds

1 tablespoon raw pine nuts (or raw sesame seeds or raw tahini)

2 tablespoons lemon juice

1 garlic clove

3/4 teaspoon coconut aminos (or nutritional yeast)

1/2 teaspoon dried dill (optional)

Cracked or ground black pepper, to taste

Water

# INSTRUCTIONS

1. Rinse, dry and plate romaine lettuce.

2. For *Almond Parmesan*, add almonds, vinegar, salt, spices and nutritional yeast (optional) to food processor or high-speed blender. Process until almonds are coarsely ground and resemble ground parmesan cheese. Set aside.

3. For *Raw Caesar Dressing*, peel garlic and add to food processor or high-speed blender with lemon juice. Process until smooth. Then add remaining ingredients and process until smooth, about 1 - 2 minutes. Add enough water to reach desired consistency.

4. Drizzle *Raw Caesar Dressing* over salad and sprinkle with *Almond Parmesan*. Serve immediately.

# Smoked Salmon Avocado Salad

Prep Time: 10 minutes

Servings: 1

## INGREDIENTS

*Salad*

2 cups soft lettuce leaves (looseleaf or butterhead varieties)

1/2 cup watercress or dandelion leaves (optional)

2 oz smoked salmon

1/2 avocado

1 sprig fresh dill

1 tablespoon caviar (optional)

*Avocado Cream Dressing*

1/2 avocado

1 sprig fresh dill

1 tablespoon lemon juice

1/2 teaspoon ground black pepper

1/2 teaspoon Celtic sea salt

1/2 coconut

Water

## INSTRUCTIONS

1. For *Salad*, rinse, dry and plate lettuce and watercress or dandelion leaves (optional). Cut avocado in half and remover pit. Dice or slice avocado flesh in peel, then scoop onto greens. Lay smoked salmon over greens.

2. For *Avocado Cream Dressing*, remove coconut flesh from peel and add to food processor or high-speed blender with enough water to reach desired consistency. Process until smooth and creamy, about 1 - 2 minutes. Strain mixture through nut milk bag and place back into blender.

3. Scoop remaining avocado flesh into blender. Add lemon juice, 1 sprig dill, salt and pepper and process until well combined and smooth, about 1 minute.

4. Drizzle *Avocado Cream Dressing* over salad. Mince remaining dill and sprinkle over salad. Dollop caviar over salad (optional).

5. Serve immediately.

# Pesto Tomato Caprese

Prep Time: 5 minutes

Servings: 2

## INGREDIENTS

1 large yellow tomato

1 large red tomato

Small bunch fresh basil

Celtic sea salt, to taste

Crack or ground black pepper, to taste

*Basil Pesto*

2 cups basil leaves (packed)

1/4 cup raw pine nuts

1/2 - 1/3 cup raw oil (coconut, walnut, almond, sesame, etc.)

2 garlic cloves

1/2 lemon (or 1 tablespoon raw apple cider vinegar)

1/4 teaspoon Celtic sea salt

## INSTRUCTIONS

1. For *Basil Pesto*, peel garlic and add to food processor or high-speed blender with squeeze of 1/2 lemon. Process until finely chopped. Add pine nuts, basil, oil and salt and process until finely ground, about 1 minute.

2. Slice tomatoes and plate in alternating colors. Sprinkle with salt and pepper. Chiffon basil leaves.

3. Spread *Basil Pesto* over tomato slices and top with fresh basil. Serve immediately.

# Cilantro Taco Salad

Prep Time: 10 minutes

Servings: 1

INGREDIENTS

*Salad*

2 cups lettuce (chopped)

1/2 cup cilantro (chopped)

1 plum tomato

1/2 small onion

1 garlic clove

1 avocado

1/2 lime

1/2 jalapeño

Paprika, to taste

Ground black pepper, to taste

Celtic sea salt, to taste

*Raw Taco Meat*

1/4 cup walnuts

2 - 3 sundried tomatoes

1/4 teaspoon cumin

1/8 teaspoon garlic powder

1/8 teaspoon smoked paprika

1/8 teaspoon ground white pepper (or ground black pepper)

1/8 teaspoon teaspoon Celtic sea salt

# INSTRUCTIONS

1. For *Salad*, rinse, dry and plate lettuce and cilantro. Reserve pinch of cilantro in small mixing bowl.

2. Peel onion and dice. Reserve 1/2 of onion in separate mixing bowl and add remaining onion to reserved cilantro. Remove seeds from jalapeño ad mince. Dice tomato. Add to onion and cilantro with squeeze of lime. Sprinkle on pinch of salt and pepper, and mix to combine. Set aside.

3. Cut avocado in half and remove pit. Scoop flesh into bowl with reserved onion. Peel garlic and mince, and add to avocado with squeeze of lime. Sprinkle on salt, pepper and paprika to taste. Mash slightly and mix with fork until well combine but still chunky. Set aside.

4. For *Raw Taco Meat*, add walnuts, sundried tomatoes, salt, pepper and spices to food processor or high-speed blender. Pulse until coarsely ground.

5. Top *Salad* with *Raw Taco Meat*, avocado and tomato mix. Serve immediately.

# Asian Shrimp Lettuce Wraps

Prep Time: 35 minutes

Servings: 2

INGREDIENTS

4 large lettuce leaves (thin, flexible ribs)

1 cup cabbage (shredded)

1 small carrot

1/2 green onion

1/2 inch piece fresh ginger

1 small garlic clove

1/2 teaspoon raw sesame seeds

1/2 teaspoon coconut aminos (or tamari or raw apple cider vinegar)

1 teaspoon raw oil (sesame, coconut, walnut, almond, etc.)


*Shrimp*

10 - 12 medium shrimp

3/4 cup lemon juice (about 5 lemons)

1 teaspoon red pepper flakes

1/2 green onion (scallion)


*Almond Sauce*

2 tablespoons raw oil (sesame, coconut, walnut, almond, etc.)

1/4 cup raw almond butter (or 1/2 cup raw almonds)

1 tablespoon lemon juice (or coconut aminos or tamari)

1/2 small mild chili pepper

Water

# INSTRUCTIONS

1. For *Shrimp*, slice green onion and reserve half in small mixing bowl. Peel, devein and remove tails from shrimp. Add to separate bowl with lemon juice, remaining green onion and red pepper. Mix to combine. Shrimp should be completely covered in lemon juice. Place in refrigerator for 30 minutes, or until shrimp are opaque.

2. Peel ginger and garlic, and finely grate or mince. Add to green onion with coconut aminos and oil. Mix to combine. Set aside.

3. For *Almond Sauce*, add oil, almond butter or almonds, lemon juice and chili pepper to food processor or high-speed blender. Process until smooth and creamy, about 1 - 2 minutes. Add enough water to reach desired consistency. Transfer to serving dish.

4. Shred cabbage and carrot and add to ginger mixture. Toss to coat.

5. Rinse, dry and plate lettuce leaves. Drain shrimp and layer onto lettuce. Top with cabbage mixture and sprinkle on sesame seeds. Roll up lettuce wraps and serve with *Almond Sauce*.

# Chicken Fries with Garlic Aioli

Prep Time: 10 minutes

Cook Time: 15 minutes

Servings: 2

INGREDIENTS

8 oz boneless, skinless chicken breast

1 egg

1/2 cup almond meal

1 teaspoon flax meal (or ground chia seed)

1 teaspoon ground black pepper

1/2 teaspoon paprika

1/2 teaspoon onion powder

1/2 teaspoon garlic powder

1/2 teaspoon chili powder

1/2 teaspoon sea salt

*Garlic Aioli*

1/2 - 3/4 cup coconut oil

1 egg yolk

2 garlic cloves

1/2 small lemon

1/4 teaspoon ground white pepper (or black pepper)

1/4 teaspoon sea salt

3 tablespoons flavorful oil  (black truffle, walnut, almond, sesame, etc.)
(optional)

# INSTRUCTIONS

1. Heat large pan over medium-high heat and coat with coconut oil.

2. For *Garlic Aioli*, peel garlic and add to food processor or blender with egg yolk, juice of 1/2 lemon, salt and pepper. Process until smooth, scraping down sides of vessel.

3. While processor or blender is running, very slowly drizzle in enough coconut oil to create thick mayo-like mixture. Drizzle in flavorful oil as well will processor runs (optional). If mixture is runny, drizzle in more coconut oil while processor runs until thickened. Pour into serving dish and refrigerate.

4. Slice chicken into half width-wise, creating twice the fillets. Try to slice at thickest portion to keep all fillets equal thickness.

5. Slice chicken fillets into long, 1/2 inch wide strips. Place strips between two paper towels and press to absorb excess moisture.

6. In a shallow dish, blend almond meal, flax or chia meal, spices and salt.

7. Beat egg in small mixing bowl. Toss chicken strips in beaten egg to lightly coat, then dredge in seasoned almond meal.

8. Carefully place coated chicken strips into hot oil and fry about 2 - 3 minutes, until golden brown and cooked through. Turn with tongs half way through cooking.

9. Drain cooked chicken on paper towel, then transfer to serving dish.

10. Serve hot with *Garlic Aioli*.

# Quick Chili

Prep Time: 5 minutes

Cook Time: 20 minutes

Servings: 4

## INGREDIENTS

1 lb lean grass-fed ground beef (or elk, bison, turkey or chicken)

15 oz (1 can) organic tomato sauce

6 oz (1 can) organic tomato paste

1 small onion

1 bell pepper

2 cloves garlic

2 tablespoons chili powder

1 tablespoon ground cumin

1 tablespoon smoked paprika (or paprika)

1 teaspoon Mexican oregano (or dried oregano)

1 teaspoon ground black pepper

1 teaspoon sea salt

1/2 teaspoon cayenne pepper

1 tablespoon coconut oil

sea salt, to taste

## INSTRUCTIONS

1. Heat medium pot over medium-high heat. Add 1 tablespoon coconut oil.

2. Peel onion and garlic. Stem and seed bell pepper. Chop and add to food processor or bullet blender. Pulse until finely minced.

3. Add to skillet and sauté for about 1 minute. Add ground beef and spices. Brown beef for about 5 minutes. Stir with whisk to break up meat well, or wooden spoon to keep beef chunkier.

4. Add whole cans of tomato sauce and paste. Stir to combine.

5. Bring to a simmer, then reduce heat to medium and cover loosely with lid to prevent splatter. Simmer about 10 minutes. Stir occasionally.

6. Use large serving spoon or ladle to serve hot.

# Dinner Ideas

## Zucchini Pasta with Sundried Tomato Sauce

Prep Time: 5 minutes

Servings: 2

INGREDIENTS

1 large zucchini

*Zesty Tomato Sauce*

2 medium tomatoes (or 3 plum tomatoes)

5 sundried tomatoes

2 tablespoons raw cashews (or 1 tablespoon raw cashew butter)

2 large garlic cloves

Small bunch fresh basil leaves

1 small fresh oregano sprig

Ground black pepper, to taste

Cayenne pepper, to taste

Celtic sea salt, to taste

INSTRUCTIONS

1. Carefully slice zucchini with spiralizer, vegetable peeler, or sharp knife. Sprinkle with pinch of salt, pepper and cayenne. Gently toss to coat and set aside.

2. For *Zesty Tomato Sauce*, remove basil and oregano leaves from stems. Peel garlic. Add to food processor or high-speed blender with tomatoes, sundried tomatoes, cashews or cashew butter, salt, pepper and cayenne. Process until smooth, about 1 - 2 minutes.

3. Transfer zucchini pasta to serving dishes. Top with *Zesty Tomato Sauce* and serve immediately.

# Zucchini Pasta with Pesto

Prep Time: 10 minutes

Servings: 2

## INGREDIENTS

1 small zucchini

1 bell pepper (or 1 carrot)

*Pine Nut Pesto*

2 1/2 cups fresh basil leaves

1/2 cup raw pine nuts

1 garlic clove

2 tablespoons raw oil (walnut, almond, coconut, sesame, etc.)

1/4 teaspoon ground white pepper (or ground black pepper)

1/4 teaspoon Celtic sea salt

## INSTRUCTIONS

1. Carefully slice zucchini with spiralizer, vegetable peeler, or sharp knife. Carefully slice carrot with spiralizer, vegetable peeler, or grater, if using. Or remove stem, seeds and veins from bell pepper, then julienne (cut into long thin slices). Set aside.

2. For *Pine Nut Pesto*, peel garlic and add to food processor or high-speed blender with basil, 2 tablespoons pine nuts, oil, salt and pepper. Process until thick, smooth mixture forms, about 1 - 2 minutes.

3. Add *Pine Nut Pesto* to veggie pasta and toss to coat. Transfer to serving dish and top with remaining pine nuts. Serve immediately.

# Zucchini Fettuccini Alfredo

Prep Time: 10 minutes

Servings: 2

## INGREDIENTS

1 medium zucchini

1 carrot (or 1 small sweet potato)

*Alfredo Sauce*

1 cup raw cashews

1 teaspoon lemon juice (or raw apple cider vinegar)

2 garlic cloves

1/2 teaspoon dried thyme

1/2 teaspoon Celtic sea salt

Water

*Walnut Parmesan*

1/2 cup raw walnuts

3 tablespoons nutritional yeast

1/4 teaspoon ground white pepper (or ground black pepper)

1/2 teaspoon Celtic sea salt

## INSTRUCTIONS

1. Carefully slice zucchini and carrot or sweet potato with spiralizer, vegetable peeler, or grater. Set aside.

2. For *Alfredo Sauce*, peel garlic and add to food processor or high-speed blender with cashews, lemon juice, thyme and salt. Process

until smooth mixture forms, up to 5 minutes. Add enough water to reach desired consistency. Set aside.

3. For *Walnut Parmesan*, add walnuts to clean food processor or high-speed blender and process until finely ground. Add nutritional yeast, salt and pepper. Process until coarsely ground and mixture resembling parmesan cheese forms.

4. Add *Alfredo Sauce* to veggie pasta and toss to coat. Transfer to serving dish and top with *Walnut Parmesan*. Serve immediately.

# Cashew Crunch Kelp Noodle Salad

Prep Time: 10 minutes*

Servings: 2


INGREDIENTS

1 package (12 oz) kelp noodles

1/2 lemon

1/2 small red bell pepper


*Cashew Sauce*

1 cup raw cashews

1/2 small red bell pepper

1/2 lemon

1 tablespoon coconut aminos (or raw apple cider vinegar)

2 large basil leaves

1/2 teaspoon smoked paprika

1/2 teaspoon ground black pepper

1/2 teaspoon Celtic sea salt

1/4 teaspoon ground turmeric (optional)

1/4 teaspoon smoked chili powder (optional)

Water


INSTRUCTIONS

1. *Soak 3/4 cup cashews in enough water to cover at least 4 hours, or overnight in refrigerator. Drain and rinse.

2. Drain and rinse kelp noodles. Add to medium bowl with warm water and juice of 1/2 lemon. Set aside 5 minutes.

3. Cut bell pepper in half. Remove stem, seeds and veins and set half of pepper aside. Julienne (thinly slice) remaining bell pepper and add to medium mixing bowl.

5. For *Crunchy Cashew Sauce*, add soaked cashews, bell pepper, juice of 1/2 lemon, coconut aminos, basil, salt and spices to food processor or high-speed blender. Process until smooth, about 2 minutes. Add enough water to reach desired consistency. Set aside.

4. Drain kelp noodles and add to sliced bell pepper. Add *Cashew Sauce* and toss to coat. Transfer noodles to serving dishes.

5. Roughly chop remaining 1/4 cup cashews. Sprinkle noodles and serve immediately. Or refrigerate for 20 minutes and serve chilled.

# Raw Walnuts Tacos

Prep Time: 35 minutes

Servings: 2

INGREDIENTS

4 large lettuce leaves (thin, flexible ribs)

1 plum tomato

1/4 red onion (or white or yellow onion)

Medium bunch cilantro

1 avocado

1/2 lime

*Taco Meat*

1 cup raw walnuts

1/2 cup sundried tomatoes

1/2 teaspoon ground cumin

1/4 teaspoon garlic powder

1/4 teaspoon smoked chili powder

1/4 teaspoon Celtic sea salt

Cayenne pepper, to taste

*Cashew Sour Cream*

1/2 cup raw cashews

1 lemon

1/8 teaspoon Celtic sea salt

3 tablespoons cup water

1/3 cup ice

# INSTRUCTIONS

6.  *Soak sundried tomatoes in enough water to cover at least 2 hours, or overnight in refrigerator. Drain.

7.  For *Taco Meat*, add soaked tomatoes, walnuts, salt and spices to food processor or high-speed blender. Process until chunky mixture forms, about 1 minute. Set aside

8.  For *Cashew Sour Cream*, add cashews, lemon juice, salt, water and ice to clean food processor or high-speed blender. Process until smooth, about 2 minutes.

9.  Chop cilantro. Dice tomato. Thinly slice onion. Cut avocado in half, then remove pit and slice in peel.

10. Fill lettuce leaves with *Taco Meat*. Scoop avocado slices onto *Taco Meat*. Drizzle on *Cashew Sour Cream*. Top with diced onion and tomato, and sprinkle of chopped cilantro. Top with squeeze of lime.

11. Fold lettuce around filling and transfer to serving dish. Serve immediately.

# Tilapia Lettuce Wraps

Prep Time: 35 minutes

Servings: 2

## INGREDIENTS

1 lb boneless, skinless tilapia fillets (or other white fish)

1 1/4 cup lemon juice (about 8 lemons)

4 large lettuce leaves (thin, flexible ribs)

1 cup cabbage (shredded)

1 small carrot

1/2 green onion (scallion)

*Cilantro Sauce*

1/2 cup raw cashews

1 lemon

1/2 inch piece fresh ginger

1 small garlic clove

Medium bunch cilantro

1/4 teaspoon Celtic sea salt

3 tablespoons water

1/3 cup ice

## INSTRUCTIONS

1. Juice lemons into medium mixing bowl. Cut tilapia into 1 inch strips. Add to lemon juice and toss to coat. Tilapia should be completely covered in lemon juice. Place in refrigerator for 30 minutes, or until tilapia is opaque.

2. Carefully slice carrot with spiralizer, vegetable peeler, or grater. Shred cabbage. Slice green onion. Set aside.

3. For *Cilantro Sauce*, remove cilantro leaves form stems. Peel ginger and garlic. Add to food processor or high-speed blender with cashews, lemon juice, salt, water and ice. Process until smooth, about 2 minutes.

4. Remove tilapia from refrigerator and drain. Gently rinse, if preferred. Fill lettuce leaves with tilapia. Add shredded cabbage and carrot. Drizzle on *Cilantro Sauce*. Top with sliced green onions.

5. Fold lettuce around filling and transfer to serving dish. Serve immediately.

# City Clam Chowder

Prep Time: 35 minutes

Servings: 2


INGREDIENTS

2 dozen live littleneck clams

1 - 1 1/2 cups lemon juice (about 8 lemons)

2 cups tomato juice (about 4 large tomatoes)

2 plum tomatoes

1 celery stalk

1 carrot

1 red bell pepper

1 green bell pepper

1/4 teaspoon cayenne pepper

1/2 teaspoon onion powder

1 teaspoon dried oregano

1 teaspoon dried basil

1 teaspoon ground black pepper

1 teaspoon Celtic sea salt


INSTRUCTIONS

5. Have fishmonger shuck clams. Or carefully shuck clams yourself. Reserve clam juice.

6. Juice lemons into medium mixing bowl. Add clams and toss to coat. Clams should be completely covered in lemon juice. Place in refrigerator for 30 minutes, or until clams are opaque.

7. Juice large tomatoes in juicer then add to food processor or high-speed blender. Or add to food processor or high-speed blender and process, then strain and return to processor.

8. Remove stems, seeds and veins from bell peppers. Cut red and green bell pepper in half. Cut carrot and celery stalks in half. Add half of each veggie to tomato juice with salt and spices. Process until smooth, about 2 minutes. Add to medium mixing bowl. Set aside.

9. Dice plum tomatoes, and remaining celery, carrot, and bell pepper. Add to tomato purée with reserved clam juice, salt and spices.

10. Remove clams from refrigerator and drain lemon juice. Gently rinse, if desired. Add to bowl and mix to combine.

11. Transfer to serving dish and serve immediately.

# Creamy French Onion Soup

Prep Time: 15 minutes*

Dehydrating Time: 6 hours

Servings: 2

INGREDIENTS

3 cups raw almond milk (or 1 cup raw almonds + 4 cups water)

1/2 lemon

1/4 cup tamari (or coconut aminos or raw apple cider vinegar)

1 tablespoon coconut aminos (or tamari or raw apple cider vinegar)

2 tablespoons raw oil or butter (ghee, cacao butter, coconut butter, almond oil, walnut oil, coconut oil, etc.)

1/2 teaspoon dried thyme

1/2 teaspoon cracked black pepper (or ground black pepper)

*Caramelized Onions*

2 onions

1 tablespoon raw honey (or 2 dried pitted dates)

1 tablespoon tamari (or coconut aminos or raw apple cider vinegar)

1 tablespoon raw oil (almond, walnut, coconut, etc.)

1/4 teaspoon Celtic sea salt

INSTRUCTIONS

1.  *Soak almonds in 1 cup water at least 6 hours, or overnight in refrigerator. Drain and pop off skins, if preferred.

2. For *Caramelized Onions*, add dates, tamari, oil and salt to food processor or high-speed blender and process until smooth. Add water to reach desired consistency, if necessary.

3. Or add honey, tamari, oil and salt to large mixing bowl and mix to combine. Peel onions and thinly slice. Add to bowl and toss to coat.

4. Prepare several dehydrator or parchment sheets and line dehydrator tray. Spread coated onion on prepared trays and place in dehydrator on 110 degrees F for 6 hours.

5. Add soaked almonds to high-speed blender with 3 cups water. Process until well blended and almost smooth, about 1- 2 minutes.

6. Strain mixture through nut milk bag, cheesecloth or strainer back into processor. Reserve almond pulp and dehydrate for almond flour.

7. Add juice of 1/2 lemon, coconut aminos, tamari, oil, thyme and black pepper to almond milk. Add half of *Caramelized Onions* and process until smooth, about 1 minute.

8. Add half of remaining *Caramelized Onions* and pulse until onions are roughly chopped.

9. Transfer to serving dish and top with remaining *Caramelized Onions*. Serve immediately.

# Salmon Tartar Stack

Prep Time: 10 minutes*

Servings: 2

INGREDIENTS

8 oz boneless, skinless salmon fillet (sushi grade)

2 limes

1 avocado

1 shallot

1 tablespoon raw oil (coconut, walnut, almond, sesame, etc.)

1 teaspoon mustard seeds (or ground mustard)

Medium sprig fresh dill

Celtic sea salt, to taste

Ground black pepper, to taste

2 teaspoons caviar (optional)

INSTRUCTIONS

1.  Have fishmonger prepare salmon fillets. Or fillet salmon and remove pin bones and skin.

2.  Dice salmon and transfer to serving dish. Top with squeeze of 1/2 lime and sprinkle of salt and pepper. Place in mold to form, if preferred.

3.  Peel and thinly slice shallot, then add to small mixing bowl. Juice whole lime into food processor or high-speed blender. Add oil, mustard seeds and pinch of salt and pepper. Process to combine, then add to shallots.

4. Or add lime juice, oil, ground mustard, salt and pepper to shallots. Mix to combine and set aside.

5. Cut avocado in half and remove pit. Dice flesh in peel and scoop into separate mixing bowl. Finely chop dill and add to avocado with squeeze of remaining 1/2 lime, salt and pepper. Mix to combine.

6. Add avocado dill mixture to salmon. Then top with shallot mixture and caviar (optional). Serve immediately.

7. *Or refrigerate 2 hours and serve chilled.

# Simple Steak Tartar

Prep Time: 10 minutes*

Servings: 2

## INGREDIENTS

10 oz beef tenderloin

Small bunch fresh parsley

1/2 lemon

2 cage-free egg yolk (optional)

2 tablespoons raw oil (coconut, walnut, almond, sesame, etc.)

1 teaspoon ground mustard (or mustard seeds)

1 shallot

1/4 teaspoon chili flakes (optional)

Ground black pepper, to taste

Celtic sea salt, to taste

## INSTRUCTIONS

1. Finely dice tenderloin and parsley. Add to bowl with squeeze of lemon and pinch of salt and pepper. Mix to combine.

2. Transfer to serving dish. Place in ring mold to form, if preferred. Set aside.

3. Peel shallot and mince. Add to small mixing bowl with egg yolks (optional), mustard, oil, salt and spices. Whisk to emulsify.

4. Top tenderloin with mixture and serve immediately. Or refrigerate 20 minutes and serve chilled.

# Macadamia Crusted Ahi Tuna

Prep Time: 5 minutes

Cook Time: 1 minute

Servings: 1

INGREDIENTS

8 oz ahi tuna fillet

1/4 teaspoon coconut oil

1/4 teaspoon dried thyme

1/4 teaspoon dried tarragon (optional)

1/4 cup whole macadamia nuts (shelled)

1 small garlic clove teaspoon

1 small shallot teaspoon

1/2 teaspoon ground white pepper (or black pepper)

1/2 teaspoon sea salt

2 tablespoons coconut oil

INSTRUCTIONS

1. Heat medium pan over medium-high heat. Add 2 tablespoons coconut oil to pan.

2. Chop macadamia nuts well. Peel and finely mince garlic and shallot. Set aside.

3. Rub top and bottom of fillet with 1/4 teaspoon coconut oil, salt, pepper, thyme and tarragon (optional).

4. Press 1/2 chopped macadamia nuts into each side of fillet.

5. Add garlic and shallots to hot oiled pan and sauté for just a second. Do not burn.

6. Carefully place fish in pan and sear 15 - 30 seconds on each side, for rare to medium rare. Carefully flip half way through cooking.

7. Transfer fillet to serving dish and serve hot with mixed greens or favorite veggies.

# Parchment Baked Salmon

Prep Time: 5 minutes

Cook Time: 20 minutes

Servings: 1


## INGREDIENTS

8 oz salmon fillet (deboned, skin-on)

6 - 8 medium asparagus stalks

1/2 lemon

1 basil sprig

1 rosemary sprig

1 teaspoon coconut oil

Pinch black pepper

Pinch sea salt

Parchment paper

Kitchen twine


## INSTRUCTIONS

1. Place large sheet pan on bottom rack of oven. Preheat oven to 400 degrees F. prepare parchment sheet.

2. Place salmon in middle of parchment sheet skin-side down and sprinkle with salt and pepper. Place asparagus stalks next to salmon. Cut lemon into thin slices and place over fish and asparagus. Rub herbs between palms, then lay basil and rosemary sprig over lemon slices. Drizzle 1 teaspoon coconut oil over salmon and asparagus.

3. Gather edges of parchment up over salmon and tie tightly with kitchen twine to form sealed pouch.

4. Place pouch directly on hot baking sheet in hot oven. Bake for 20 minutes.

5. Remove from oven and carefully transfer pouch to serving plate. Carefully open pouch to release steam.

6. Serve hot.

# Snack Ideas

## Sausage And Peppers

Prep Time: 5 minutes

Cook Time: 10 minutes

Servings: 4

INGREDIENTS

4 Italian sausage links (pork, chicken, etc.)

1 white onion

1 bell pepper

INSTRUCTIONS

1. Heat large skillet over medium heat. Add 1 tablespoon coconut oil.
2. Peel onion. Stem and seed pepper. Roughly chop onion and pepper. Slice sausage into 3/4 inch slices.
3. Add sausage to hot oiled skillet and sauté about 2 minutes. Then add onion and peppers. Sauté about 8 minutes, until sausage is cooked through and browned.
4. Serve hot.

# Spicy Chicken Bites

Prep Time: 5 minutes

Cook Time: 10 minutes

Servings: 4

INGREDIENTS

8 oz boneless skinless chicken

1/2 cup almond meal

1 teaspoon flax meal

1 teaspoon paprika

1/2 teaspoon cayenne pepper

1/2 teaspoon red pepper flakes

1/2 teaspoon ground black pepper

1/2 teaspoon sea salt

1 egg

1 jalapeño pepper

2 garlic cloves

2 oz organic spicy brown mustard

Coconut oil (for cooking)

INSTRUCTIONS

1. Heat a medium skillet over medium high heat. Lightly coat pan with coconut oil.

2. Slice chicken into 1x1 inch strips. Arrange slices between 2 sheets of parchment and pound with kitchen mallet or rolling pin to flatten slightly. Place flattened pieces between two paper towels to absorb excess moisture.

3. In a shallow dish, blend almond meal, flax meal, dry spices and salt.
4. Add egg , jalapeño and peeled garlic to food processor or bullet blender. Process until fairly smooth. Pour into shallow dish.
5. Dip chicken pieces into jalapeño egg, then dredge in seasoned almond meal.
6. Carefully place coated chicken pieces into hot oil and fry about 2 minutes, until golden brown and cooked through. Turn with tongs half way through.
7. Drain cooked chicken on paper towel, then transfer to serving dish.
8. Serve hot with spicy mustard.

# Simple Guacamole

Prep Time: 5 minutes

Cook Time: 5 minutes

Servings: 4

INGREDIENTS

2 avocados

1 shallot

1 small tomato

1 bunch cilantro

Half lime

2 teaspoons paprika

1/2 teaspoon ground cumin

1/2 teaspoon ground black pepper

1/2 teaspoon sea salt

INSTRUCTIONS

1. Peel and finely dice shallot. Dice tomato and cilantro. Add to small mixing bowl.
2. Slice avocados in half, pit, and scoop flesh into bowl. Add 1 teaspoon paprika, 1/2 teaspoon cumin, 1/2 teaspoon black pepper and 1/2 teaspoon salt.
3. Mash avocado and mix ingredients well with fork. Transfer to serving dish and squeeze on juice of half a lime. Sprinkle with remaining teaspoon of paprika.
4. Serve immediately. Or refrigerate 30 minutes, and serve chilled.

# Green Deviled Eggs 'N Ham

Prep Time: 5 minutes

Cook Time: 10 minutes

Servings: 4

## INGREDIENTS

8 eggs

1 avocado

1/2 teaspoon ground black pepper

1/2 teaspoon salt

2 oz natural ham

2 tablespoons fresh dill

## INSTRUCTIONS

1. Bring medium pot of lightly salted water to boil. Gently add eggs to hot water with tongs and cook about 8 - 10 minutes.
2. Drain eggs in colander and cool in cold water.
3. Crack shells and peel eggs. Cut eggs in half lengthwise and scoop out yolks into small bowl. Arrange whites on platter with center hollows facing up.
4. Mash avocado, salt and pepper with egg yolks until smooth. Dice ham and dill, separately.
5. Scoop avocado blend into each egg white hollow and sprinkle with ham, then dill.
6. Refrigerate about 20 minutes. Serve chilled.

# Pigs In A Blanket

Prep Time: 20 minutes

Cook Time: 15 minutes

Servings: 4

## INGREDIENTS

1 package(26 count)  nitrate-free/nitrite-free mini hot dogs

3 egg whites

1/4 cup almond flour

1/4 cup coconut flour

1 tablespoon cold coconut oil

1/2 teaspoon baking powder

Pinch garlic powder

Pinch sea salt

2 oz organic mustard

## INSTRUCTIONS

1. In separate medium bowl, mix almond and coconut flours with baking powder. Cut-in cold coconut oil, then add pinch of garlic powder and salt.  Mixture should be crumbly.  Refrigerate 15 - 20 minutes.

2. Preheat oven to 400 degrees F. Line sheet pan with parchment or lightly coat with coconut oil.

3. Whisk egg whites in medium bowl until white and frothy, just before soft peaks develop.

4. Gently fold egg whites into refrigerated flour mixture until just combined.

5. Flatten 1 level teaspoon of dough into a rectangle in your fingers. Place one sausage in middle of dough wrap it around the sausage. Repeat with remaining sausage and dough.

6. Place wrapped sausages on prepared sheet pan and bake about 15 minutes, until dough is golden brown and links are heated through.

7. Serve hot with mustard.

www.ingramcontent.com/pod-product-compliance
Lightning Source LLC
Chambersburg PA
CBHW070437290526
45791CB00005B/2010